CW00591392

BUTTERFLYING

A POCKET-BOOK
FOR MENTAL HEALTH

BUTTERFLYING

A POCKET-BOOK
FOR MENTAL HEALTH

ANNE PRESTON

with a contribution by

EMMA HARDING

CROFT PUBLICATIONS

2013

First published 2013
by Croft Publications
on behalf of Anne Preston
Flat 2, 48 Thrale Road,
London, SW16 1NX

© Anne Preston 2013

All rights reserved. No part of this book may be
reproduced, stored into a retrieval system,
or transmitted in any form
or by any means (electronic, mechanical,
photocopying, recording or otherwise)
without the written permission of the author.

ISBN 978 0 955126 8 1

Typeset by Croft Publications
The Croft, 8 St James Meadow,
Boroughbridge, YO51 9NW
www.croftpublications.co.uk

Printed and bound by
Smith Settle Printers and Bookbinders Ltd
Gateway Drive, Yeadon, LS19 7XY

Contents

*This book is dedicated to those who
did not make it.
May they Rest in Peace.*

Acknowledgements

My thanks go to Patrick Holford for giving me permission to quote from his book *Optimum Nutrition for the Mind* (Published 2003 by Judy Piatkus Ltd).

I also wish to thank my two long-suffering and patient 'Technical Advisers', my good friends and neighbours, Maureen Nawrat and Michael Collins, and Cat Nawrat and Eve Kelley, for permission to use their photographs, also to Emma Harding for kindly contributing the chapter entitled *Recovery*. I would not have been able to complete this book without the professional support of Dr Peter Hughes and Dr Rob Chaplin. Thanks also go to my cousin, Ken Cothliff, who introduced me to my publisher, Terry Nicholson.

I would not have succeeded in finishing this book were it not for the love and support I have received from my good, kind and generous friends in London, Brighton and Ireland who have looked after me in so many ways. They know who they are. And last but by no means least, heart-felt thanks and love to my beautiful daughter, who has been with me at my worst and hopefully now, at my best.

Some names have been changed in order to achieve anonymity.

Introduction

'Capricorns grow younger as they grow older'. This pronouncement was made by my dear Great-Aunt Peggy when she heard the news of my arrival into the world in the January of 1944. Britain was in the grip of a terrible war with Germany, but I was fortunate enough to be born near Manchester and conditions there were not as bad as in London and the South of England where bombing of civilian areas was common.

I enjoyed a very happy and carefree childhood, surrounded for the first five years of my life by a loving and generous extended family of Grandparents, my dear mother and assorted aunts and uncles who were happy to spend time making my life very secure and full of enriching experiences, especially a deep love of books to which I was introduced at an early age.

The only person missing from my childhood was my father, who was posted to Egypt with the RAF when I was a year old. He returned for a short spell of leave when I was three and I remember he took me up for a pleasure flight around Southport, but he did not return to England permanently until I was rising five.

Of course he loved me, but I do wonder whether my later mental health problems were connected with the lack of my father's presence during my formative years.

However I did well at school, despite a couple of primary school moves and grew up in the Shropshire countryside and around the Malvern Hills. My sister was born in Shropshire and I was so proud of her. Being just five when she arrived I was able to be the 'big sister' and enjoyed playing this role immensely.

I won a scholarship to a girls' public school in Worcester at ten, and proceeded to shine at various subjects, particularly English and Latin.

When I was fourteen my father was posted to Hampshire and my parents gave me the choice of moving with them to Hampshire and changing schools or living with my best friend's family during term-time and staying at my school in Worcester. My friend's parents had very kindly offered this option and I decided to take it, as I was settled and happy at my school, and had stayed with them several times already and enjoyed being with them.

Looking back, I can see how crucial this decision was to my development, not only education-wise, but also in the development of my personality.

My friend's family was very different from my own. Whereas my life at home up to this point had been well-ordered and slightly bourgeois, my new family was intellectual, untidy and a little chaotic but we always had regular and plentiful meals, and my friend's parents treated me as one of their own daughters. In fact, they had lost their eldest daughter when she was ten and I always hoped I could perhaps, in some small way, make up for this tragedy, although no pressure was put on me to do so. I would sometimes help my friend's mother do the washing-up after supper, as her own daughters did not help her and she would often talk with me about her job as a teacher at the local secondary modern school.

I realise now that I am something of a chameleon, as I tend to adapt easily to my surroundings. This was what I did at the end of every school term, when I went home to wherever my own family was based. I believe the seeds of my mental illness took root about this time. Naturally there had to be come some rebellion against this situation. At first it would be small comparisons between my father and my friend's father who was a donnish, retiring type, but who kindly took my side in the rare event of me getting into any trouble. My own Dad, being a military man and used to having his own way, did not take kindly to my budding socialist views, being a die-hard Tory. We would have fiery arguments when I would provoke his short temper, and my poor Mum, who was the peace-keeper in the family, found herself in the middle of this difficult situation, as well as having two younger children to look after.

I did well at school and it was suggested by my teachers that I try for Oxbridge, which meant staying another year at school. However, I could not wait to leave this rather cloistered existence and procured a place for myself at Manchester, the only university which would would accept me, aged seventeen.

Already I was drifting. I told those who asked me, why I wanted to go to university, that I had gone 'for the life', and indeed that was probably more important than my French and Russian studies.

I managed to pass my my first year exams and set off for France where I had found a summer job coaching three children in a French family. It was my first visit to France despite the fact that I already spoke quite fluent French. The family hired a chalet in the French Alps each summer and this place was to become my Waterloo. As soon as I stepped into the house I felt uncomfortable although I hardly registered this uneasy feeling consciously.

The children were bright and I particularly enjoyed working with Henri, the eldest, who spoke excellent English and with whom I could have discussions about religion and philosophy on our walks in the beautiful alpine countryside near Allevard. He was only thirteen but exceptionally intelligent.

Gradually as the weeks passed I became withdrawn and my inner world began to fragment. I continued teaching the children each morning, but their mother, Madame, whom I rarely encountered and who did not eat with the rest of the family, had shown me a cutting from an English newspaper. Apparantly, in Birmingham, a scientist working with rats had caught bubonic plague. In my rapidly deteriorating state of mind, I started to imagine that everyone around me was gripped by the plague. Although to those with whom I had contact, I presented as a reasonably normal person, inside my mind was in chaos and confusion.

I realised I had to get home as soon as I could. During a rare conversation with Madame I told her I must return to England. I was soon on a train bound for Calais. Somehow I boarded the ferry for Dover and my guardian angel must have been working overtime, as by now I needed some good Samaritans to come to my aid. I had noticed passengers leaving the saloon and in my psychotic state of mind, thought they were going to throw themselves overboard, as they were suffering from the plague.

Friends later told me they were amazed that I had managed to travel across France and board the ferry in my weak and confused state but I believe my guardian angel was working overtime to protect me.

A young couple took me under their wings. They must have realized I was unwell and I had told them that the rest of my family was on holiday in the Isle of Wight. Karen and Cornel were two good Samaritans and took me home with them to Kingston-upon-Thames. I remember they were artists and not much older than me. They called their doctor who admitted me to Brookwood Psychiatric Hospital.

This was to be the beginning of my journey through mental distress and *Butterflying* offers a distillation of the elements in life which have helped my recovery, be they people, animals, gardens, yoga or music or more ethereal influences *i.e.* my Christian Faith.

CHAPTER 1

The Matter of Faith

'Be Still and Know that I am God'

This sounds an easy enough thing to do and is good advice if we can quieten our minds and bodies down enough to contact this inner silence. However, if you are in mental turmoil, distress or depression this is not so easy to achieve.

When I was 18 I had my first breakdown and was hospitalised and sedated for two weeks so that when I tried to get out of bed and walk my legs gave way beneath me. I also had six ECT treatments and the interesting part is that I thought I had passed over into heaven and that the weeping and wailing I could hear from the adjoining ward was people on the earth in travail, which indeed it was, but I was still part of it.

After about three ECT treatments I realized I had not passed over to the other side, but that my mind had led me down some hitherto unknown and bizarre pathways. For someone brought up with a conventional Church of England background this came as a profound shock to my system and to my soul. My lifes journey had taken a very different turn from that generally expected of a promising undergraduate. I believe the diagnosis was 'nervous exhaustion' but there was a bit more to it than that.

I had a so-called 'boyfriend', who had told me before I left Manchester at the end of the summer term that he was coming to France for the summer but he made no contact with me and, looking back, I think I was hoping throughout my stay that he would contact me but he didn't. I think this contributed to my depression.

We finally arrived at Dover and caught the train to Victoria. Then we went by Green Line Coach to Kingston where my good Samaritan lived. I do remember noticing the colour of the bus. Karen and Cornel lived in Queens Road, Kingston-on-Thames. I remember their flat was comfortable and bohemian.

They gave me a meal and then they must have called their doctor because I hazily remember him coming to the house and saying I would have to go to Brookwood Hospital near Woking. Presumably I travelled by ambulance as Karen and Cornel did not have a car.

And now I regress back to the day I was confirmed. I was fourteen years old and the confirmation service took place in Worcester Cathedral where I was at school.

Two things stand out in my mind about that day. The first is that I said to my godmother, Aunty Katherine, who was there at the cathedral for me, 'I have to give the Bishop a bob' – she replied 'why do you have to give him a shilling?' ('bob' was slang for the old shilling, and we were both laughing 'no, I mean I have to curtsey to him when I have been confirmed')! The other memory is of my headmistress, Miss Roden, saying to us girls, 'try to remember one thing that is spoken during the service and which has significance for you'. As we were filing out of the cathedral past the great organ which was booming out some triumphant music, I remembered the words of the Bishop: 'redeemed and forgiven'. They will stay with me forever.

On my return to the UK following my first breakdown in France, I was transferred from Brookwood Hospital which was in Surrey, to the Herts and Essex hospital in Bishops Stortford near my parents home and soon I was visited by the local curate, Tim, who was the most saintly and kind man and with whom I fell in love. He did not realize this – at least I do not think so, but he was the person through whom I found my faith and which has remained and grown – despite some severe setbacks, largely due to depression, and on which I have built my life.

Tim to me was Christ-like – an example of a human being who has devoted his life to the service of others and through whom I had a glimpse of our Lord. As so often happens with God – he arrived just when he was needed. I was at a very low ebb and my life had fallen apart – I felt different from other people because of my illness, but later I realized this was all part of a long and difficult process to understand the needs of the mentally ill, and to be able to put myself into their shoes. These early experiences would stand me in good stead when I came to work at Springfield (Psychiatric) Hospital, both as librarian and later as an advocate and as a volunteer on the chaplaincy team.

Tim wrote me some very encouraging letters after I left hospital and I started attending the local church but, as with anyone's faith, mine needed nourishing, and it was not until I was married to David that I found another Pastor like Tim.

David was in the throes of a breakdown himself when I found a church and a Pastor who could offer me the help I needed. This time the help came from – the Lutheran Church in Harlow, Essex, where David and I and our small daughter had made our home. The church was close to our house and Pastor Val Hennig was its leader. Val was a very approachable and friendly man, as well as being strong in the faith and very understanding of life's problems. I managed to get David to come with me to church and after a short time we decided to be confirmed into the Lutheran Church. The fundamental tenets of the Church were no different from the Protestant Church of England, but the way the Pastors were chosen was not the same. There was also a different hierarchy in the priesthood from the Church of England.

I eventually found myself elected chairman of the Ladies Guild at the church, and was very busy finding speakers and running meetings. The church was a simple, modern whitewashed building with no adornments and there was a large congregation which consisted mainly of young families as Harlow was a New Town. I did find the fellowship with these people very supportive and my faith was strong despite David suffering further breakdowns and being in and out of work. Sophie was christened here and I became a Sunday School teacher. When our marriage finally broke down, I left this church and once again I was in the wilderness. Looking back I can see how important it is to nourish one's faith. By leaving the fold, so to speak, I was cutting myself off from my source of nourishment and I did not bother to replace it with another.

Looking back on my second marriage, I think I was depressed most of the time and I even had a suicide attempt, and I do believe things would have been different if I had found a supportive church and Pastor with whom I could share my problems. Eventually, I met a lovely elderly chaplain at Springfield Hospital and he became a great source of strength for me. In fact I met and got to know a series of elderly chaplains, at the hospital, all of whom in their own way, helped me through these difficult and loveless times.

Charles Goslin came out of retirement to help at Springfield Hospital Church. He was already in his eighties when I met him but he was sprightly and walked everywhere. He had a keen sense of humour and a great love of books and that was how I first encountered him, as he visited the library at the hospital where I worked and we fell into conversation. We became firm friends and when, after several years of service at the hospital, he became ill with cancer, I visited him in St. Thomas Hospital. I had a very unusual experience at this time. I went to bed as usual and fell asleep. Later in the night I was aware of two dark-skinned gentlemen in the room. Immediately I knew they meant death. Then I felt myself leave my body (very easily and quickly) and I found myself entering a place filled with light and who should be standing there but Charles! I thought this meant my own death and I was very concerned about Sophie but I just said to Charles 'I don't recognise this place' and he replied (typically) 'philosophers never take notice of their surroundings!' A few seconds later and I was back in my body. Two or three days later I heard Charles had died and I realized it was his death I had foreseen.

This experience helped me to realize that 1) it is easy to leave the mortal body behind and 2) I did not fear death anymore.

As time went on a new chaplain arrived at Springfield – David, with whom I was eventually to work closely. I started to help him in small ways in the church such as laundering the church linen and we had many conversations on all sorts of topics – I found him interesting and amusing – he had been a Franciscan monk but, after much contemplation, decided to ask the then Archbishop of Canterbury to be freed from his vows of poverty, chastity and obedience and to return to life outside the monastery. So here he was at a large London psychiatric hospital, suggesting that I train as a Lay Reader at Southwark Cathedral, so that I could officially be a volunteer on the Chaplaincy team at Springfield. It did not take long for me to make up my mind – it involved a three year course on a Thursday evening and I quite relished the prospect of studying again – it was a challenge which I was happy to take up.

On Thursday evenings I would drive to Southwark Cathedral and, with about twenty other trainee lay readers, would study such characters as Iraneus, the Synoptic gospels and St. Paul, practice delivering a good sermon and discuss such issues as homosexuality and spirituality in the present-day world. It was stimulating, encouraging and mixing with other students was fascinating for me – we went on retreat to a convent in Wimbledon one weekend and spent much of the time in silence. I felt like a naughty school-girl when I was passed a note by another student asking me to accompany him for a walk on Wimbledon Common!

At the end of the three year training there was a licensing ceremony in the Cathedral where we were proudly presented to the then Bishop of Kingston and wore our blue stoles for the first time. My parents and some close friends were in the congregation as we processed up the aisle to be licensed.

My ministry was to be divided between Springfield Church and St Pauls Church in Streatham. My first sermon was on Advent Sunday at St Pauls and I used the theme of doors opening and closing in our lives. One member of the congregation at St Pauls who was to become a friend and who was later ordained gave me some good feedback on the content of my talk and I felt great. It is always encouraging to hear positive things from one's peers.

But I have to confess that I felt at this time my spiritual home was at Springfield. I loved driving up there on Sunday mornings and the wonderful fellowship that existed amongst the staff and patients who came to the church. We would bring some of the geriatric patients down in wheelchairs and they were so grateful. One morning a young patient came running into the church where the service was already in progress. She flung herself in front of the altar and then stood up and asked David if he would use the sliced loaf of bread she was carrying, for communion. He, not in the least bit fazed, gently took the loaf from her and blessed it and said he would use it for communion. She went and sat down with the rest of the congregation and the service proceeded without further ado. This is what I loved about Springfield services – there was so much spontaneity and true emotion that you felt you were connecting with something very special and far closer to God. The Peace was always a precious time – the old people would kiss you and hold on to you and often I thought this was the only real human touch they experienced during the whole week.

My sermons at Springfield were deliberately short but they usually packed a punch and one Sunday I was preaching on forgiveness and cited the example of Bette Lynch, one of the characters in *Coronation Street* who had forgiven her screen husband for having an affair. I knew most of the congregation followed 'The Street' and indeed they clapped and cheered. For me it was a great moment.

In 1988, I became involved in a relationship with a man who was an atheist. He was comfortably off to say the least and initially we got on well. I was going through a difficult time in my library career and he was supportive and understanding. I had reached a turning point in my career and decided, on health grounds, as I had developed asthma, to take early retirement from the library service. I moved down to Guildford to live with him. About this time my mother became ill with cancer and I devoted much of my time to nursing her through the final stages of this awful disease. Once again I had cut myself off from my source of spiritual nourishment and when my mother died in February 1990 I slid into a bad depression.

I had moved down to Guildford to live with Fred and this was really the start of what was eventually diagnosed as bi-polar (manic depression) disorder. I was going through the menopause, my mother was no longer around – she who had been such a source of support and strength to me. And I was involved in a relationship with a man who did not hold to the same belief and value systems as I did.

I think all these factors combined pushed me to have drastic mood swings which took the form of winter depressions lasting from about September to April followed by manic summers.

During these depressive periods I felt far from God, sometimes even completely abandoned by him and my faith dwindled. Life became a real struggle – as with most depressive people, the mornings were the worst time and it was an effort to drag myself out of bed – as the day progressed the depression diminished somewhat, and by the evening I felt reasonably normal. Fred – showed some understanding of my predicament and I became quite dependent on him emotionally and for company. I often drove up to London to spend time with my best friend, Anne and her two young sons. I felt comfortable with old friends who accepted me as I was, but I found difficulty in socialising with people I did not know well. Fred bought a house in West Sussex and I moved there with him. I did attend the village church but my faith was hanging by a thread and often my life seemed meaningless. Materially I was better off than I had ever been in my life but that was not why I had moved in with Fred. I had wished to escape from London and its pollution and frenetic way of life and yet I had found myself in another difficult and challenging situation from a spiritual point of view.

After a couple of depressing winters I found a mentor in a local parish priest who was also a psychotherapist. He agreed to see me on a regular basis and I found great solace in our talks together. He pointed out that I was living in a 'guilded cage' and eventually I decided in the summer of 1994 that I had to leave Fred. I had made this decision during the previous winter but knew I would have to wait until I had the impetus of the summer mania to make the break.

I succeeded in leaving him, but landed up in Graylingwell Psychiatric Hospital in Chichester and once again I experienced total abandonment and separation from God. I was sectioned and injected, against my will, with a drug which made me totally paranoid and physically ill. After a couple of months incarcerated in this hell hole, my car keys were returned to me and I drove into Chichester to attend morning service at the cathedral. I thanked God so much that morning that I had my freedom once more. But my high mood led down into another trough and I became depressed as the summer faded and autumn days drew in. I finally left Graylingwell in September and returned to my flat in London, much against my wishes – I longed to stay in Sussex but I did have my supportive daughter and good friends in London and God guided me back for what would prove to be a long stay.

I cannot say that my faith was strong at this time. One morning I was feeling pretty desperate and decided to attend the Church of England church at the end of the road. After the service we were offered someone to pray with if we needed it and I found a delightful gentleman in a wheelchair sitting beside me. He introduced himself as Arthur and prayed with me. I was in tears but I felt great empathy flowing from Arthur and felt comforted by his kind and understanding words. Several years later when I started attending this church regularly, I found out that Arthur was in the latter stages of multiple schlerosis and I would visit him at home whenever I could. He had been a surgeon before he became ill and I could but dwell on the awful irony of this – a loving and clever doctor struck down by a terminal illness and having to be completely reliant on other people, especially his courageous and caring wife.

I was to endure a spell in another psychiatric hospital in South London as my depression worsened and I was plagued by more 'O' attacks. However, I did attend the hospital church occasionally and it provided some comfort during a very rocky period. This was the hospital where I had worked for so long as librarian and on the chaplaincy team, and I could not help feeling humiliated by my present predicament. It was yet another lesson – I could not always be the giver to those less fortunate than myself – sometimes I had to be the receiver. The conditions on the ward, which was locked, were very bad. One day at lunchtime a fight broke out as lunch was being served – tables were being overturned and hot food thrown about – it was terrifying and we girls took refuge in our dormitory until things had simmered down. I was frequently offered illegal drugs and even sex for money. This was indeed the devil's domain and you needed survival skills to endure it.

However, better things were on the horizon. After Christmas 1994, I left the ward and attended instead the Day Hospital which meant I was living independently again. The atmosphere here was more like a college and I made some good friends.

During this period I embarked on a spiritual search. I started attending the local Spiritualist Church where I frequently received 'messages' supposedly from 'the other side'. Some of these I definitely discounted, as the events predicted did not happen. Sometimes I received comforting advice and occasionally the events predicted did happen. I continued to attend for some time but eventually I felt that 1) I should not put my trust in mediums – there is an infinitely greater power, and my earlier understanding of the Bible as God's word, expressly warned against dabbling in this sort of divination. 2) I did not find the 'worship' side of the services uplifting and 3) I did not have to come away from a church service truly feeling I have worshipped my maker. This is generally through music, prayer and silence in order to be in God's presence more fully.

I started visiting the Buddhist Temple in Wimbledon. It is a Thai Temple and is attended mostly by the Thai community in London. Here, in the beautiful and peaceful gardens and woods, I found real peace. On Sundays during the summer I would often attend the lunch provided in the garden of the monastery and sometimes meditate with the monks in the temple. On other occasions I would simply sit under my favourite tree in the grounds and commune with nature. I can honestly say I have found more peace here than anywhere else in London. The kindness and gentleness of the monks and the Thai people is truly amazing and I am often drawn back to Wimbledon for a 'top-up' of this inner peace.

As I write I am about to take a flight to Thailand, a largely Buddhist country and a place I have wanted to visit for several years. However, I have returned to my Church of England roots and often attend the local Church of England church at the end of my road. This quest for peace and a closer relationship with God is a continuing and lifelong journey. Every morning I try to remember to pray for opportunities during the coming day to serve my Lord and frequently my prayers are answered – often in very surprising ways! You never know whom you will encounter at the bus stop, or who will come knocking on your door – that for me is part of the adventure which my quest for truth offers – it is nothing to do with the dogma and pomp of the church – it is to do with a life lived to the full, seizing opportunities to show a glimpse of Christ to other people and never forgetting that we are all part of one great universal family.

Recently, I have been given the opportunity to get to know a Muslim family. They have received me into their home and treated me as an honoured guest. I am truly humbled by this experience and wish to get to know them better. Understanding and tolerance start in small ways like this. There is real love in their household and I feel I am being shown yet another facet of the Almighty. We should be emphasizing the similarities between our faiths – not the differences which divide and bring hatred amongst nations and individuals.

There is a rich seam of culture in all the great faiths and we should try to educate our children both at home and in school to have a greater knowledge and understanding of the culture surrounding the great faith systems, pointing out that the Islamic culture grew out of the Judaeo-Christian tradition. The great houses of Damascus which are adorned with fabulous mosaics and fountains are only one of many examples of Islamic art and architecture which flowered in the 16th century and followed on from the Christian tradition. In the area of Spain around Seville and Cordoba the Muslims and Christians lived side by side and one has only to look at the great cathedrals and mosques in that area to see how the two faiths flourished contemporaneously.

The positive aspects and similarities of all the great religions should be taught to the next generation who will have to deal with the legacy of our mistakes and misunderstandings. The world is changing rapidly – great migrations of peoples are happening as I write, and we are constantly having to adapt to new situations and living in a multi-cultural society, particularly in the big cities. It is by individual relationships with people from other cultures that we make our judgements and perceptions but we also need a knowledge of where they are coming from – what makes them 'tick' and how we can best build bridges in our local communities. Here in Streatham one Christian's full-time job is to do just that – build bridges with the Muslim Community through visits by Christians to local mosques and vice versa and by personal friendships between people of the two faiths.

My search for truth and knowledge is a life-long one, an ongoing adventure but my role in all this is very simple – I dedicated my life to relieving suffering in whatever ways I could, when I left the big house in Sussex. That promise has not changed – I am a servant of Christ and I hope I will continue to find opportunities to carry out this task in whatever way I can as long as I am able.

Chapter 2

Support Systems

Family and Friends and other Sources of Support

During the times that I suffered with mental health problems I was very fortunate to have some very supportive and understanding people around me. The first and perhaps most important figure in my support system was my dear mother Marion. Although my mother had two younger children to look after, she never failed to visit me when I was in hospital at the age of eighteen after my first breakdown in France, and she supported me when I had to spend time at home afterwards. I will never forget the shock in her face when my parents first visited me in the dreadful old psychiatric hospital in Surrey where I had landed up after returning from France. I believe my mother came close to a breakdown herself at that time, but somehow she found the inner resources to cope with a new and very disturbing and difficult situation.

My mother's way of helping me was to chat to me about everyday things as if everything was normal but this seemed to gradually bring me back to some sort of normality and it was my mother who suggested, when

I finally realized I could not complete my degree, that I try to find work at the local library. I was drifting at this point and needed a pointer for my life and this guidance from my mum was exactly the right direction for me at that time. I plucked up the courage and rang the library and was offered an interview and was accepted onto the staff at Harlow Central Library.

I eventually qualified as a professional librarian and this work enabled me to support my daughter when I became a single parent and it was very rewarding, particularly when I became librarian at Springfield Psychiatric Hospital.

My Aunty Katherine, my mother's elder sister, who is now ninety six years old and an amazing person, has also always been there for me when I have been unwell. Aunty Katherine, who is one of my godmothers, has shown great empathy and love and has often provided me with financial help when I have needed it. This constancy from my family including my daughter, Sophie, who has had to support me in some very difficult situations which I would not have wished upon her, has greatly helped in my recovery process. Sophie would talk me through my 'O' attacks when she was only a teenager and had a great way of dealing with my sometimes strange behaviour. Added to this she has also had the unpleasant task of getting me admitted to hospital several times and this cannot be easy for anyone. Mental distress can place a heavy burden on children when they sometimes have to take on the role of carer at a young age. More help is needed in this area for young carers. Sophie had the additional burden of a father who had mental health problems and although he was not living with us, it placed further pressure on her young life. I am hopeful now that I will not be plagued any more with mental distress. I do not wish for Sophie to have any more burdens laid upon her. There is so much to do in life and I feel I have wasted a lot of time being ill. Now it feels like I finally found my true identity and can live a fulfilled life and also help others along the way.

There are many other people who have been there for me in times of trouble. My best friend Anne has always been a tower of strength – when I returned to London in 1994 and was suffering with bad depression I did not want to live on my own, Anne offered to have me live with her family. Fortunately I managed to get my life together again and did not need to take her up on her generous offer, but it was so good to know I had such a supportive friend. Anne says I have always been there for her in a crisis and I do believe firmly that friendship is a matter of give and take – we never know when difficult times are going to loom on the horizon and a network of loving and supportive family and friends is so important.

I was lucky enough to meet a lovely man in 1995 who saw me through some very black periods when I was plagued by 'O' attacks and depression. I believe I would have been in hospital if it had not been for Phil. He was the most unselfish man with whom I have had a relationship and was, I'm sure, a gift from God. We parted in 2000 but I will never forget Phil's great generosity of spirit and his buoyant nature which never let me down. Some days, when my mood was really black, Phil would take me out with him on his delivery rounds and it did give me an uplifting of spirits to be driven out of London and to see the countryside and nature in all its glory. An understanding and caring partner, in my opinion, is the single most important factor in the recovery process.

My best friend Anne, whom I have known for 28 years has also had mental health problems and I think this has been an important factor in our friendship because we can understand to some extent how the other is suffering although the nature of our mental distress has been different. Anne is now managing an advocacy service and her great ability to solve difficult problems and understanding of mental health issues has given her service an excellent reputation – she has helped so many people in difficulty and deserves recognition for her hard work.

As I wrote at the beginning of this chapter, there are people with mental distress who do not have a supportive circle of friends and family. One of the main problems which faces these souls is isolation as there is still a stigma attached to this illness and they can find themselves marginalized by society, and this only adds to their misery. Also it should be made clear that there are different degrees of severity of mental illness. Some people are able to hold down a job, despite suffering from depression, for example. Somehow they manage to drag themselves out of bed and get to work. I can speak from experience – this is not easy but often the nature of depression is that it is worst in the morning and alleviates as the day wears on and if this initial effort can be made it is worth the torture of getting going in the morning.

I was fortunate to obtain a part-time post, shortly before I retired, at a womens' drop-in in South London. I had initially been invited to do a head and shoulder massage demonstration for the women at the drop-in but as so often in life, I was pointed in this direction in order to do more work.

I loved helping at this very caring and mutually supportive centre and made some very good friends, both with the members and the other staff. We ran a poetry group and even published an anthology of our work – we painted on glass and produced a gorgeous wall-hanging with each square sewn by a different woman – this was exhibited in a centre in Mitcham, Surrey. One memorable Tuesday we had a 'Makeover' Day. One member was a hairdresser and did the womens' hair. Another was a make-up specialist and one of the younger members photographed the gorgeous results. It was indeed a transforming experience and one of the best days ever in my working life. I also taught some yoga to the women and they really enjoyed it.

The importance of day centres and Sunday lunch clubs cannot be underestimated – they provide a relaxed and non-judgmental environment for those who might be lonely (especially at weekends) and they can often produce lasting and supportive friendships amongst the members. Although they are often run on a shoe-string budget, they provide great value for money and in terms of improving mental health, they are invaluable.

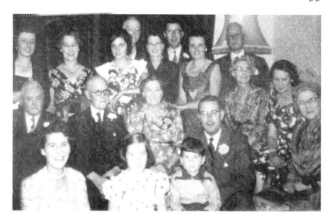

My paternal grandparents' golden wedding anniversary.

Chapter 3

Nutrition and the Mind, including Herbal Medicine and Vitamins

We are, obviously, what we eat. This is a physical fact, but, what we eat and drink, can also affect our mental state. We see the effects of food particularly in children – they can rapidly become hyperactive if there are synthetic colourings in their diet. We have all heard of the dreaded 'E' numbers and if we are careful we will check our groceries to make sure they do not contain these additives. So a surplus or a lack of certain minerals and/or vitamins can affect our mental state.

However Patrick Holford, founder of the Institute of Optimum Nutrition recommends, as a result of much research on the subject, that each patient should have a tailor-made programme which addresses diet and supplements to bring them back into balance.

Those who suffer with a mild form of SAD syndrome (winter depression) can boost their mood by taking St. Johns Wort (Hypericum perforatum) in capsule form or in tea bags, if the depression is relatively mild. The herb has fewer side effects than tricyclic anti-depressants such as imipramine. A dose of 300mg three times a day should help to alleviate the symptoms of winter depression. It does however take about two weeks to work but this is less time than most anti-depressants. It is not yet known exactly how St. Johns Wort works but a large research project in the USA should soon reveal a lot more about the workings of this herb. The main advantages of taking it are – you can still drink alcohol without adverse reactions, there are no withdrawal symptoms if you stop, it does not inhibit your libido and it enhances sleep and dreaming. However, St. Johns Wort does not interact well with lithium and should be avoided if you are prescribed lithium. SAD syndrome is related to lack of sunlight and low mood can be boosted by daylight bulbs which are readily available in the shops now – also by light boxes, but these are more expensive. It is very common for your mood to be lower in the winter months when the sun is at its lowest and, particularly in Britain, we experience many gloomy, grey days. I know also from my own experience that I feel worse if I am unable to sit outside in the garden in the sunshine which is often the case from about November till April. It is better to go for a brisk walk at least once a day than hibernate in the house during the winter months.

Depression can be a result of repressed anger and often sufferers have buried this emotion so deeply that they are almost unaware of it and wonder why they feel so low. Psychotherapy can help in some of these cases- by unravelling the past where perhaps a dream has not been realized or a relationship has failed and the emotional fall-out has not been dealt with, can often alleviate the problem. With cases of deep depression the patient may need psychotherapy and some interim medication.

Patrick Holford in his book *Optimum Nutrition for the Mind* writes, 'there are often two sides to feeling blue – feeling miserable and feeling unmotivated and apathetic. The most prevalent theory for the cause of these imbalances is a brain imbalance in two families of neurotransmitters, the molecules of emotion. These are:

Serotonin, which influences your mood and Adrenalin and Noradrenalin, made from dopamine, which influences your motivation. All the major anti-depressant drugs are designed to influence the balance and function of these neurotransmitters.

Women are three times as likely as men to experience low moods. This is because, as research has shown, that women have lower serotonin levels than men. In addition to a lack of tryptophan (which is especially rich in turkey, oats, fish, cheese and eggs etc.) there are six main reasons for serotonin deficiency:

Not enough oestrogen (in women)

Not enough testosterone (in men)

Not enough light

Not enough exercise

Too much stress, especially in women

Not enough co-factor vitamins and minerals'

Tryptophan has been found to lead to an increase in the synthesis of serotonin and therefore it is recommended that low mood requires 1g and up to 3g for actual depression.

Here are five ways of eating 500mg of Trytophan:

Oat porridge, soya milk and 2 scrambled eggs.

Baked potato with cottage cheese and tuna salad.

Chicken breast, potatoes au gratin and green beans.

Wholewheat spaghetti with bean, tofu or meat sauce.

Salmon fillet, quinoa and lentil pilaf and green salad with yoghurt dressing.

If you are depressed you may be low in folic acid. Patrick Holford recommends a dose of 1, 200mg per day if you suffer with severe or chronic depression. Folic acid is only available in supplements of 400mg in the UK therefore you should take 3 tablets per day. He also recommends taking Vitamin B6 at 200mg per day. These nutrients help the production of the hormone serotonin in the brain which boosts our mood.

Other mood boosters are the Omega 3 fats which help boost the brains neurons. The higher your intake of Omega 3 fats the better your brain produces serotonin. Low cholesterol can also be a contrbutory factor in depression. The best way to ensure that you get adequate cholesterol in your diet is to eat herring, tuna, sardines and mackerel.

It should be noted that we do not all react well to higher doses of folic acid. Some people have high blood histamine levels and overproduce histamine. High dose folic acid stimulates the production of histamine in these people and makes the depression worse. This was discovered by Dr. Carl Pfeiffer the founder of Princeton (USA) Brain Bio Centre and is an example of how each person has a unique body chemistry so that what works for one individual does not necessarily work for another. When histamine levels become too high chronic depression can result.

Two famous examples of probable high histamine types are Judy Garland and Marilyn Monroe who both committed suicide. Vitamin C should be taken by supplementing 2 mg per day. Foods which are mood enhancers include tomatoes, brazil nuts and turkey (which contains tryptophan).

Niacin, part of the B vitamin group (B3) is synonymous with nicotinic acid. As a co-enzyme it assists in the breakdown and utilization of fats, proteins and carbohydrates. Lean meat, eggs, liver, fish and wheatgerm and even beer have appreciable amounts. In its role as co-enzyme, niacin helps in the oxidization of sugars and is essential to proper brain metabolism. In 1966, Pfeiffer and Iliev discovered the possible role of histamine in schizophrenic patients and noted that niacin in conjunction to a maximum of 3 gm daily with other vitamins, raised blood histamine and thus helped to relieve such symptoms as paranoia, hallucinations and other disperceptions.

Niacin should be taken with equal doses of Vitamin C. It' should be taken after meals to minimize flushing and nausea. Dosage can vary from 50mg to a maximum of 3 gm per day. The best response is from schizophrenic patients who are low in histamine. The response of those who are improved is frequently much better than those on tranquillizers alone.

An amino acid, tryptophan, can be converted into niacin by body chemistry. Thus, niacin may be obtained from tryptophan-containg foods such as poultry, eggs, meat and dairy products. Some people can obtain their daily requirement of B3 from their diet but those schizophrenics who can benefit from it may need much larger doses taken in tablets.

Niacin therapy (niacin used in conjunction with Vitamin C) heralds a new age in the biochemical treatment of schizophrenia and yet how often do British psychiatrists presribe it? It is far more effective when used with tranquillizers than tranquillizers used alone and permits the use of lower doses of these powerful drugs with consequently a reduction in side effects.

In my opinion schizophrenic patients are frequently prescribed too much medication – often resulting in unwanted side-effects such as weight-gain and even eventually, diabetes.

When I was working as an advocate a common problem brought to us by clients was the unwanted side effects of anti-psychotic medication. Young female patients particularly suffered loss of confidence and anxiety over their weight gain and added to the still existing stigma attached to mental illness. This often made for great unhappiness and poor self esteem and who was benefiting? The obvious answer is of course the pharmaceutical companies who are making vast profits out of peoples' misery. Many doctors benefit from the inducements offered by the drug companies, such as 'team-building' holidays abroad for the psychiatrists and their teams.

The proposed – European Legislation restricting the sale of herbal remedies will give the big drug companies even more power.

Chapter 4

Yoga –My Antidote to Depression

I first started practising yoga during the early eighties when a friend invited me to attend a small yoga group in her house. We met once a week and almost immediately I started to feel the benefit of the practice. I needed approximately one hours less sleep each night and I found if I did a fifteen minute set of asanas (postures) in the morning before going to work I had more energy during the day. Of course we all looked forward to the 'relaxation' at the end of the session, but I found this was a good balance for my body and mood. Also the breathing exercises associated with the asanas are very beneficial, especially as I suffer with asthma.

After a few months my friend introduced me to another yoga teacher, Daya Murti, who was a yogi. We started to attend yoga classes at her centre, Yoga Kutir in Mitcham, Surrey and I found Daya Murti a constant source of inspiration and a shining example for the art of yoga. Daya Murti looked at least twenty years younger than she actually was and always gave the impression of being very youthful and indeed her mind was in excellent shape and she has now written many books on yoga. I heard recently from another yoga teacher that she has found love and gone to live in Australia – I wish her all luck in the world.

Of course yoga is a very ancient practice, first expounded in the Bhagavad Gita. Sri Krishna teaches Arjuna directly the Perfection of Yoga. It is a complete way of life enhancing mind, body and spirit and needs daily attention *i.e.* practising the asanas and breathing exercises as well as a having a right attitude of mind. We are always thinking that by changing our situation we will overcome our mental agitation and we are always thinking that when we reach a certain point, all mental agitation will disappear. But it is the nature of the material world that we cannot be free from anxiety. However, by practising daily the asanas, breathing and right thinking, we can reduce our anxiety levels and if we really persevere

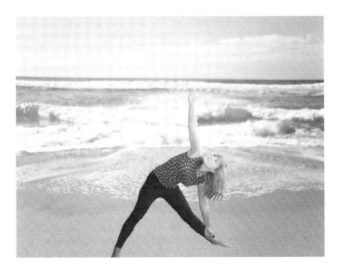

Cat practising Trikonasana.

we may reach the stage where we are completely free of it and can view the world with equanimity regardless of what is thrown at us, whether it be other people's anger or other emotions- indeed something to strive for.

 In his book entitled *The Perfection of Yoga His Divine Grace*, A. C. Bhaktivedanta Prabhupada says, 'we should regard everything in the same light whether it be a stone, gold or a crystal.' In other words we should not put worldly values on objects. This is another difficult exercise, especially when applied to people. Naturally we make judgements about people with whom we come into contact, but we should try to remember that we are all God's children and everyone has a right to respect. This is particularly true with regard to those with mental health problems who are still often regarded as second-class citizens through no fault of their own. Hopefully, as a more enlightened attitude towards those suffering mental distress emerges, we may not feel the stigma as much, if at all.

During the early nineties I suffered with a lot of depression, particularly in the winter months. I found that just about the only activity I looked forward to was my yoga practice. By doing a routine every morning this was an anchor in an otherwise rather grey and choppy sea. I practised the asanas I had learnt with Daya Murti and one day she telephoned to see if she could visit me. I felt very honoured and we spent a happy time together. I still try to do a daily routine even though, fortunately I have not suffered with depression for several years.

More recently I worked at a Drop-in Centre for women with mental health problems living in the community – I was asked to do a yoga class with those women who wished to learn more about yoga which produced some very positive feedback.

In 1990, I was lucky enough to spend a holiday in India and we travelled to the north to Rishikesh in the foothills of the Himalayas where the Beatles spent time in the ashram (Yoga Centre) with the Maharishi in the sixties. Rishikesh had an atmosphere all of its own – it was full of saffron-robed monks with begging bowls and you felt the spirituality of the place immediately – of course it has been commercialised since the sixties but there was still the unique aura peculiar to India and which draws people back again and again.

In the cold crisp morning mountain air I practised my asanas and felt at one with the people and with nature. One Monday morning we walked beside the Ganges – it has its source high up in the Himalayas and flows swiftly through this region where you can see people bathing and washing their clothes in the cold water. After a couple of miles we came to a small village bustling with life and noticed amongst the shops one called 'The Himalayan Emporium'. It was only a tiny store but crammed full with all manner of goods. The people were very friendly as was the case wherever we went in India and of course wanted to sell us items of clothing etc. I was happy it was Monday and I was not working in London but instead was breathing in the pure and healthy mountain air by the Ganges river.

I have practised yoga in quite a few different places but it always brings that sense of well-being and calm especially if one is stressed or low in spirits – I am still attending a class where I find other people who also wish for a better quality of life and we are very fortunate to have a great teacher who constantly inspires and teaches new ways of attaining that ultimate goal – to become a true Yogi!

Chapter 5

Art as Therapy

I have always loved looking at pictures – even as quite a young child I can remember looking at the pictures of Rupert Bear and his friend Algy the Pug in the *Adventures of Rupert Bear*. Rupert always wore a striped scarf and checked trousers – I do think I was born with a photographic memory although this was knocked for six when I had ECT when I was eighteen. Sometimes even now I can vividly picture a face or event in my minds eye.

At school my marks for art were way below those for intellectual subjects, although I usually could picture what I wanted to paint in my mind, it rarely, if ever, turned out as I wanted. My best friend at school was very artistic and I could never emulate her and I felt a bit inferior in this respect. My mother used to talk about Aunty Dora, my great aunt, and tell us how she could not stay in a room if it was decorated in certain colours – I feel much the same way and as I get older I need harmony in every aspect of my life. Not least in colour schemes. Colour does affect our moods – I remember attending the newly decorated office of my psychiatrist – the room was painted a vivid lime-green – hardly the colour to calm anxious patients!

When I first visited the then Tate Gallery in London aged about twenty one I was pretty amazed. Up to that time my only experience of classical art had been a postcard of Leonardo's 'Last Supper' which I had bought to illustrate an essay on the Renaissance for my history course. When I sat my university exams in Manchester in the Whitworth Art Gallery in the early sixties all the pictures were covered over – presumably so that the students would not get any inspiration from them!

I continued to visit art galleries from time to time and became fascinated by the life of Van Gogh – did he become crazy from sitting out painting in the blazing sun in the South of France? How did he survive the harsh life in the Borinage – the potato-eating region of Belgium where he lived with the peasants and drew and painted frenetically? In 1993 I was fortunate enough to spend a holiday in the South of France and we visited Arles where Van Gogh and Gaugin had lived briefly during 1888. Unfortunately their house (The Yellow House) had disappeared but I soaked up the atmosphere of the place and was very moved to arrive one evening at dusk at St. Remy, the hospital where Van Gogh had been cared for during 1889-1890. It was still a place of healing and very peaceful with lights flickering in the evening gloaming and irises growing in the garden. Apparently Van Gogh suffered with psychomotor epilepsy which is characterized by short attacks during which the patient suffers intensification and distortion of perception and emotional states. I felt glad that this poor tormented genius had finally landed in a place of tranquillity and was cared for by understanding people.

My neighbour, when I worked as librarian at Springfield (Psychiatric) Hospital, was an art therapist, Chloe, whose department was next door to the library. Chloe, I discovered, lived in the next road to me and we became firm friends. The work of the art therapy department was very important – patients could come here and express their emotions in painting and drawing and they could talk to the art therapists who were highly trained in this area.

Chloe used to visit the locked ward once a week and here she found Sean, a patient who had not spoken for months. He was an artist himself and a very good one. Chloe helped him to paint and draw again and after a year of being silent Sean began to speak again. This is just one example of the healing that art therapy can bring and it is often far more effective than heavy doses of drugs.

Until I retired in 2001 I did not consider I could paint, let alone sell any work but something compelled me to enrol in an art class at Tooting (South Thames) College and I found myself loving every minute of it. It was a class of varied abilities and experience but one of the joys was to view other students' paintings at the end of the session and discuss each others' work. We had a young but very inspiring teacher, Jane, who had recently left art school. Jane taught me the rudiments of oil painting, a medium which I found suited my style. I was also fortunate to meet up with an old friend, William, with whom I had lost touch. At this class we enjoyed comparing notes on our work and getting to know the other students.

I attended the class at Tooting for a year and all this time I was also practising oil painting at home. I became very interested in the paintings and drawings of Matisse and started to copy some of them. I love his masterly use of colour, his subject matter and his innovative use of minimal lines to convey (usually) female figures. Painting is such a pleasure and I can lose myself in the work for a morning or an afternoon. For me the most exciting part of the process is mixing the colours – you never quite know what the result is going to be and oils are very versatile.

In early 2002 I mounted a small exhibition in the Babish Café in Tooting with the help of my friend Guy who had also made and painted the frames for the paintings. I did not make any sales but consoled

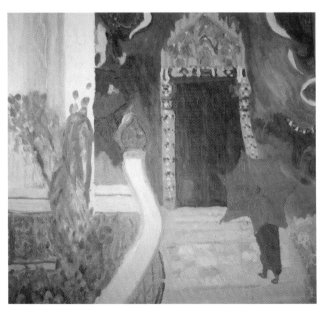

Buddist Temple in Thailand, author's painting.

myself with the thought that many artists do not have immediate financial success. Neverthe less I was keen to make a sale and painted on.

During 2007 I had a visit from Sean who has kept in touch all these years and he asked me whether I would sell him my copy of Matisse's 'Pink Geraniums' which was hanging on my wall. I felt a pang of loss in my heart – could I part with this painting into which I had put so much effort and love? But I knew the answer was 'yes' and after all I had always wanted to sell a painting! Sean departed happily carrying the painting and I had made my first sale!

A few months later another friend asked me if I would paint her an abstract and I was happy to do so. You feel so honoured when someone actually requests a work. I sold another Matisse copy to friends in Berlin in 2007 and ended the year on a high note.

I have now started to have greetings cards printed from some of my paintings and they have sold well and of course I love sending them to friends and family on birthdays and other occasions.

I really believe my painting has helped my recovery from bi-polar disorder – maybe it has something to do with releasing creativity into a painting which might otherwise find a manifestation in a 'high' – it is certainly something worth considering.

My latest project involves an exhibition of some of my original paintings at a concert by Philharmonia Britannica in February 2008 – I was so pleased to be asked to do this by the conductor of the orchestra, Peter Fender.

Recently I have started visiting the psychiatric hostel on my road and I have started painting with a group of the residents. They have produced some really interesting work and it is good for all of us to paint together and explore our creativity. I do look forward to Thursday mornings and our sessions together.

As far as I am concerned there are no hard and fast rules in art, except of course that blue and yellow make green etc, and so often people say 'I can't draw or paint' when in fact they may not have done so since schooldays – it is such a good therapy and should be offered in all psychiatric hospitals and anywhere else in the community serving users – it is a universal form of communication, as is music and should never be under-rated. Vive Matisse!

Chapter 6

Nature and her Power to Heal

Following on from the previous chapter I would like to say something about the healing power of the natural world. I spent most of my childhood in the country and took for granted the beautiful landscape around Malvern and Shropshire. My friends and I were able to cycle off for a few miles and explore the countryside and take a picnic with us – all this when we were only about ten years old. These days children would probably not have this carefree existence but we can still enjoy the natural world in other ways.

Many people live in flats in the cities and have no garden – even if this is the case it is still possible to grow herbs and other plants indoors. It is so exciting to plant bulbs (e.g. tulips, hyacinths or daffodils) in pots in October or November and see these plants flower, often in time for Christmas, or just after, when we are often at our lowest ebb – January and February are not easy months to survive but the joy derived from growing your own flowers is tremendous.

It is now the beginning of March and a beautiful sunny warm day, especially after the cold wind we have been experiencing for the last few days. I went into the garden at about nine o'clock and I did my yoga and taichi exercises outside as I always do (unless it is pouring with rain) and then – bliss – lying in my hammock for about fifteen minutes just enjoying the warmth and peace of the garden. A pair of coal tits came and sat in the tree under which the hammock is slung. I would recommend anybody to try and sling a hammock either between two trees in the garden or somewhere in the house. Its gentle rocking motion is very calming and beneficial – it is almost like being a baby again and being rocked in your mother's arms. (Habitat stocks a good selection of hammocks.)

I have noticed that people who work close to the soil do not often have mental health problems although there are exceptions – Monty Don of *Gardeners World* has spoken openly about his winter depressions and bravely

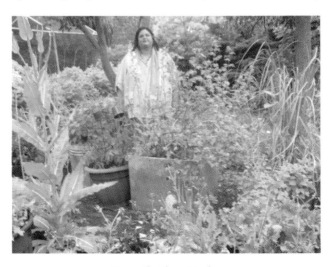

Eve in the Share Garden.

carries on with his work despite this handicap. If you do suffer in this way I can recommend walking near trees – this could be in the park or out in the countryside or just in your own garden. And of course hugging trees is very powerful – I have noticed that different trees have different energies – one is calming, another uplifting. My advice is get to know your local trees! If you live in the city just getting out into the nearest green space can help to lift your mood. Running or jogging is also a good way of helping depression as the endorphins produced by the exercise help lift the depression.

It is interesting to observe the changing seasons and how they affect us and the birds and animals and plants around us. Personally I think my favourite time is April – the end of winter and fresh life springing up all around. The weather can also be quite warm and sunny – I have even acquired a bit of a tan whilst just pottering around the garden during April!

At Springfield Hospital in South London there is a gardening project run by the charity 'Share' and staffed by three gardeners who are assisted by service users living in the community.

I visited the project on a warm June morning to talk to the staff and take some photographs of this beautiful oasis set in the middle of a densely-populated area of London. The garden covers approximately two acres and includes two polytunnels (one for vegetables and one for flowers), a pond stocked with goldfish, some colourful and well-planted beds, plenty of seating and some very old trees dating back to Victorian times when the garden was first used as an airing court for male and female patients. Jenny who runs the project told me they are now growing vegetables for use in the kitchens and it seems things have come full-circle as in the early days of the hospital the patients helped in the garden growing vegetables for consumption in the hospital. Apparently Hospital Trusts now have more awareness of their carbon footprints.

Plants, both flowers and vegetables, can be bought at this project and are not as expensive as those in garden centres. I bought some courgette and tomato plants – I shall grow them in pots in the garden but they could equally easily be grown on a window-sill inside the house. Courgettes produce fruit throughout the summer and are very easy to grow. Tomatoes need feeding with special tomato food and will also keep producing fruit throughout the summer. Other vegetables that are easy to grow are radishes, lettuce, spinach and marrows.

The therapeutic value of gardens such as this cannot be underestimated and even while I was there some service users from the drug-addiction ward came to visit and were very impressed with the peaceful atmosphere and imaginatively planted surroundings.

As we become more and more aware of the need to reduce our carbon footprint, the benefits of growing our own food and just having a space to indulge our need to be around nature in whatever form, will hopefully, become more a part of the healing process for those suffering with mental distress. It is to be hoped that there will be many more projects like the one at Springfield, which has already been part of this process for many people.

Chapter 7

Complementary Medicine and its Role in relieving Mental Distress

My first experience of the healing effect of complementary medicine took place at Yoga Kutir, a yoga centre I was attending in South London during the eighties. After our yoga practice our teacher asked me to massage her feet – she probably needed someone's touch and I was privileged enough to be asked. I worked instinctively, gently rubbing the soles and tops of her feet and also the ankles – when I had finished she thanked me and told me I should train as a reflexologist.

I had been considering a change of career and was at a crossroads in my life and I decided to act on Daya Murti's advice. At that time I was still working as a librarian but the training at the International Institute of Reflexology was at the weekends so I was able to do both. I qualified as a reflexologist in 1989.

About this time I moved to Guildford and gave up working as a librarian. I started practising as a reflexologist and eventually set up in business in a hairdressing salon in Guildford – I had also trained in Indian head and shoulder massage by this time, so offered both therapies. I often had clients referred from the hairdressers downstairs and found myself treating a variety of ailments including stress headaches (the head and shoulder massage is particularly effective in helping this problem), back problems and arthritis to name but a few. I was very privileged to have a female client for head and shoulder massage who told me she had been raped and I was the first person to touch her

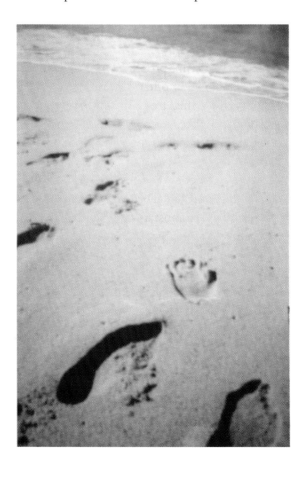

since this terrifying experince. I enjoyed this work very much and people always seemed to feel better after a treatment. However I was renting my room six days a week and found I was not making enough profit to continue, so after a few months I started working from home. I was supplementing my income from temporary jobs as I realized it is difficult to make a living as a complementary therapist alone.

I became involved in working with those suffering with HIV whilst living in Guildford and gave reflexology to some clients with this problem. I have found over the years that patients will often want to talk about their problems whilst being treated and I have even had patients in tears whilst I have been working on their feet. Somehow touch can release often long-buried emotions.

During the nineties I attended a conference in London concerning Mental Health and Complementary Therapies. It was a most inspiring and informative occasion. I met, amongst others, Patrick Holford,

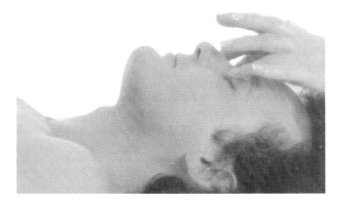

author of the book *Optimum Nutrition for the Mind*, who spoke on Nutrition for Depression and Peta Trousdell who had worked as a reflexologist in Brighton with women suffering with depression and had very good results – in some cases the need for anti-depressants was reduced and the general well-being of the women was improved.

I have treated many clients with mental health problems ranging from schizophrenia to depression, and I can honestly say they have all felt better after a treatment, whether it was reflexology or head and shoulder massage.

It is not uncommon for clients to cry during a reflexology treatment and again I feel privileged to have a small part in their recovery from often deeply buried emotional experiences. The cathartic nature of complementary medicine is not to be under-estimated. I strongly feel that there should be a part of the psychiatrist's training which includes these therapies and a more holistic approach in general for those seeking to enter the psychiatric profession.

More recently I treated a client who wished to get pregnant and thought reflexology might help. She had had a miscarriage the previous year. After three treatments she was indeed pregnant and very happy! She has recently given birth to a beautiful baby boy.

As I have mentioned head and shoulder massage can help stress headaches and related problems – when I was practising in West Sussex a woman telephoned me who had had a headache for six days, and asked whether I could help her? I said I would try and she came immediately to my house and I gently massaged her for half an hour. By the end of the session her headache had completely disappeared.

Other forms of hands-on therapies are shiatsu – very good for releasing energy blocks (I did a short course in shiatsu and found it most beneficial) and of course osteopathy which I have received several times when I have had a back problem. Usually my back has been put right in a couple of sessions. Osteopaths have a long and intensive training and are experts with any problem related to the spinal column.

Some psychiatric hospitals offer massage and other complementary therapies on the NHS. As these treatments can often reduce the need for medication it is to be hoped that this holistic approach to alleviating mental distress can be more widely offered to patients, both in the community and in hospital.

Chapter 8

The Healing Effects of Music

I first felt the upliftment and inspiration which can come from listening to a piece of music – in this instance Beethoven's *Pastoral Symphony* – when I was eighteen and recovering from my first breakdown at home with my family in Hertfordshire. Looking back I think I was still psychotic but this was masked by a surface normality, which I managed to convey to the world – in fact I still had the remnants of my religious delusions in my head. However, I felt inspired enough to write a fairly long poem whilst listening to the strains of the 'Pastoral' – so reminiscent of those happy days in the country when I was a child in Malvern.

The second piece of music to which I wrote a poem was Elgar's *Enigma Variations* – bringing even more memories of Malvern, as Elgar had written it whilst living there. It conjures up for me the undulating Malvern Hills where I often walked and climbed as child in those carefree days before I became ill.

Of course music other than classical can lift one's spirits. I remember the first time I heard Helen Shapiro singing and how her voice resonated with something inside me which I had probably never expressed before

– a certain confident stridency which I certainly lacked at sixteen years old.

And then there is the soothing effect of a lullaby sung to a child to put it to sleep – this soothing sensation can be felt by anyone – in the Bible David's mood was softened by a harp-player – I can vouch for this as I met a Celtic harp-player whilst on holiday with my aunt in Llandudno a few years ago. The strains of Michael Richard's playing echoed through a busy shopping arcade and I knew I had to buy his CD, *Cadeucus*. It has

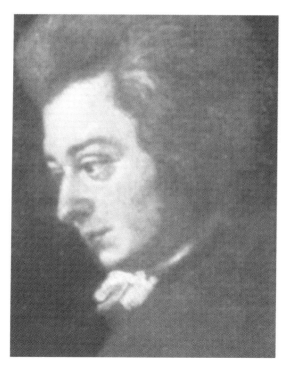

Wolfgang Amadeus Mozart (1756-1791).

brought me many hours of pleasure and often calmed my mood.

There is a phenomenon known as the 'Mozart Effect' which describes the healing and uplifting quality of Mozart's music and I have to say that if I am feeling a little low in spirits or it is a grey day, I only have to put on a Mozart CD to feel better and more buoyant in spirit.

A recent article in the *Independent* entitled 'The Medical Maestro' reported improvements in patients suffering a rare form of epilepsy while exposed to Mozart's K448 piano sonata for ten minutes a day and a 'Mozart Effect' has also been linked to behavioural and other changes, including stress, depression, arthritis pain and foetal development. I personally believe Mozart had a 'direct telephone line to God' and that his music is divinely inspired. Mozart did not have an easy life – he was dogged by money worries and did not enjoy good health but despite these difficulties he was able to rise above them and produce music which is as fresh and joyful today as when it was first written over 200 years ago.

Music Therapy is sometimes offered in psychiatric hospitals and this can only have a beneficial effect – the release of emotions through music is very therapeutic and the opportunity to beat a drum or rattle a tambourine can surely be a fine way of letting go of sometimes long-suppressed feelings. I think this therapy should be offered in every hospital – it could reduce the need for drugs and raise patients' spirits and provide a much-needed chance to make music. Unfortunately this type of therapy is not always prioritised when the budgets are being drawn up.

When I am at home either working or resting I usually play 'Classic FM' or 'Radio 3' on the radio. Both these stations play classical music and 'Radio 3' often has talks and interviews with conductors or performers. The radio is like a companion who never argues or complains! I prefer it in general to the television and of course there are always CDs – then you can choose your favourite music – whatever suits your mood. London's 'Magic' Radio station plays mellow popular music and 'Smooth FM' also tends to soothe your mood. 'Classic FM' has recently brought out a CD *Music for Babies* which includes some lovely Mozart pieces. Yes, even babies respond to music and even before they are born, still in the womb they can be lulled or aroused by certain melodies.

I have friends who have formed a concert party called 'Up Tempo' who visit elderly people living in nursing homes etc. and sing and play for these senior citizens who would not otherwise get the opportunity to hear live music. The upliftment often experienced by the elderly in response to Gershwin and other song writers is very noticeable. An afternoon spent in this way can go along way to improving the quality of life for these souls who often have happy memories of the tunes and melodies of another age.

Music is a universal language and can break down barriers of culture, beliefs and prejudice and offer a common enjoyment of its delights wherever it is played or sung – what better way to promote mental and emotional well-being?

My two favourite places to sing are 1) In Church – Preferably the old rousing hymns such as 'And did those Feet in Ancient Time Walk upon England's Green and Pleasant Land' or more modern sacred songs such as *Amazing Grace* and *Lord of the Dance* or 2) In the bath, where I can pretend I am an opera diva singing Handel's 'Didst you not hear my Lady go down the Garden Singing' or 'Thine be the Glory, Risen conquering Son!'

I know how healing and up-lifting singing in a choir can be, and recommend finding one if you desire to express yourself by singing – and it can help depression and make the spirits soar!

Chapter 9

Pets and their Therapeutic Value

My love affair with cats started when I was aged about seven years and living in Worcestershire. I used to walk past the garden at the end of our road on the way to school and one day there was a mother cat with her kittens playing in the garden. I just knew I wanted one of those kittens. I gradually wore my father down by continually begging him to allow me to have a kitten and of course in the end he gave in and I was taken up to our neighbour's house to choose one.

I settled on an adorable black and white bundle of fluff whom we called Tiny, for obvious reasons. I can still recall the long summer days in the garden at Eastwood Road playing with Tiny and I'm sure my young sister Abbie, who would have been about two and would also have had some input. I was very much the 'big sister' and would probably have supervised Abbie's activities! I remember one epic occasion when my mother realized there was a rat in the coal-shed and decided to put Tiny in there with it to finish it off. There was the most horrendous hullabaloo for some time and finally Tiny did her worst and the rat was killed.

Tiny lived to a ripe old age and since her there has been a succession of feline friends including Alpha

– the black cat that my mother adopted whilst living in Cyprus, and then when I got married we adopted Nerdi, who was brought to us on New Years Eve (she was named after the Scottish form of the 'last day' of the year), and Tuesday who was brought to me on a freezing cold February day in Harlow and who hid behind the coke boiler because she was so cold. All these cats had their individual personalities and enriched our lives with their affection and amazing ability to relax and help us relax – if you have trouble with stress in your life, a cat can only help matters. If you live alone they are wonderful companions and you will get the best welcome when you arrive home. As Katrina Smythe writes in her little book, *Your Cat – the Boss* – 'If a cat has decided to love you there is not a great deal you can do about it'!

Whilst I was working at Springfield Hospital I took home two kittens who were 'living rough' in the hospital grounds, a brother and sister as it turned out, although we thought at first they were both boys and called them Laurel and Hardy. Fortunately we had christened the female Laurel so her name remained. Sophie adored these two characters and played endless games with them. One day I found Sophie and her schoolfriend kneeling on the floor and getting the cats to jump over 'fences' made of upturned books as in a gymkhana! Sadly Hardy was run over on our busy road when he was only three years old and Laurel died of cancer a year later. It is such a sad time when you lose an adored pet and I have found that the best way of dealing with such a loss is to get another animal as soon as possible.

Taking care of a new member of the family does help the healing process, in my experience, although not everyone would want to do this and you may want to wait a while before taking on a new pet.

After Laurel's death we heard that a school friend of Sophie's whose father was a priest at Westminster Abbey had some kittens for whom they were looking for homes and we duly drove up to the Abbey and chose a pure white kitten whom we named Sanchia.

Again we derived so much pleasure from this character who was not perhaps the most brainy cat but who was gorgeous to look at and play with. When Sophie had departed for university and I had met a new man, Sanchia moved in with the new man before I did, and strangely enough he also had a white cat – the two cats being male and female were fine living together, mostly ignoring each other and getting on with the feline business of eating and sleeping and relaxing.

When my relationship with this man finished I left Sanchia with him as he had a big house and garden in the country over which Sanchia presided and he was very fond of her, particularly as his own dear cat had been run over on the main road which bordered our garden.

On my return to London after this relationship I was very depressed and Sophie and her then boyfriend kindly offered to take me to Battersea Dogs Home to find another cat. Almost immediately we spotted a beautiful tortoiseshell in a large cage named 'Maggie'. I knew she was the one I wanted and we managed to claim her and Sophie and her boyfriend duly paid the twenty five pounds necessary to bring her home. This was the best Christmas present I could have wished for. 'Maggie' was apparently three years old and had been brought to the Dogs' Home with a litter of kittens. She had been spayed at Battersea and now needed plenty of TLC. I was only too happy to oblige. We called this darling feline Petrushka and she is now sixteen and into her second kittenhood. She has been my faithful companion for thirteen years and I cannot really imagine life without her although I know she will not last forever. Petrushka is very sociable with humans and loves it when I have visitors and she has a new lap to sit on. She has been much photographed and my latest project is to attempt to paint her portrait – I'm sure I could never really do her justice – my 'Empress of Streatham' is just not reproducible but I will try.

I have only talked about cats so far but of course any pet is an enhancement to your life, be it a dog or a hamster or a ferret – they never argue or complain and if they are anything like Petrushka they are at your side through all the trials and tribulations of life, a constant source of fun and consolation.

During my time in Sussex when I was practising head and shoulder massage a dog was brought to the house. The poor animal had run headlong into a tree whilst chasing a rabbit and had injured its head. The vet had suggested the owners try head and back massage for their pet and they duly carried him up the stairs to my healing room as he could not climb the stairs on his own. I gently massaged his head and ran my hands along his back and he lay quite happily on my rug whilst

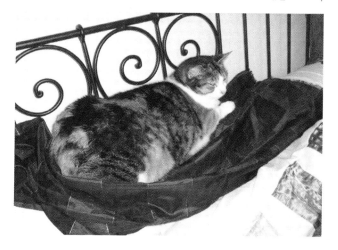

Petrushka on velvet cushion.

I intuitively worked on him. The third time the owners brought him he walked up the stairs on his own! I felt so privileged to have helped this lovely dog get back on his paws!

But this healing process works both ways and animals have healing powers – they can be a channel for healing just by sitting on your lap – I know people who have said they felt better when Petrushka was sitting on their lap and sometimes when I have been really sad or upset Petrushka has come right up to me and even made little noises (of sympathy, presumably). We should not underestimate the power of the animal kingdom to help in the healing process.

Chapter 10

Sex – The Ultimate Pleasure

I first experienced the delicious feeling of sexual desire for a man with my first boyfriend, when I was sixteen, and we were travelling on a bus one sunny afternoon in the summer of 1960. We were kissing, something I had done before but this was different, reaching a level which could have easily led to us getting off the bus and finding somewhere to make love. However, my boyfriend was quite restrained and although I think I would have happily given way to my desire, we stopped at kissing. Don't forget this was in the very early sixties when contraception was little talked about or generally used, and I think the risk of me getting pregnant was probably uppermost in my boyfriend's thoughts.

From about the age of fifteen I had masturbated but again these practices were little talked about. My mother, bless her heart, had given me a little pink book at fourteen about *The Facts of Life*. She was obviously very embarrassed and I never discussed the contents of the book with her. Fortunately my best friend's mother had been a midwife and was much more willing to discuss these 'Facts' with us and we prided ourselves on our knowledge of female biology and other related matters.

I actually lost my virginity in Geneva when I was eighteen and was raped. I must add that I was in a psychotic state when this event took place. I would not normally have gone home with a complete stranger whom I had just met in a cafe. Although at the time this did not appear to affect my sexuality, and indeed I came to enjoy sex and give birth to my daughter, the rape affected me psychologically much later in life – I think because, again it was not discussed at the time, and the aspect of fear, particularly, came to haunt me for many years after this traumatic event.

To return to the pleasures of sex, I remember distinctly the marvellous moment when my first husband and I experienced orgasm simultaneously for the first time. To hold each other afterward was such a loving and intimate experience, I cried with joy – this was what marriage should be about but these are rare and precious moments. It shows how rare, when I can only recall this particular experience once in my marriage.

Since my twenties I have had four comparatively long relationships, including a second marriage, but during my early sixties I experienced the best sex I have ever known with a wonderful man with whom I was friends for two years before we became intimate. I had never before waited so long before making love to someone and it was worth every minute of the wait. When we finally consummated our relationship it was like coming home – I knew him so well and yet there was still more to come – getting to know his body as well as his mind and with the ease the familiarity of our friendship offered, the intimacy became very precious. At first we did not have full sex *i.e.* penetration, but pleasured each other by touching and stroking but he rarely climaxed (his wish).When we did finally have full sex, and again it was worth waiting for, somehow this gradual build-up intensified the pleasures of our love-making and we both said how every time it was different – we seemed to find something new each time and often surprised each other with our inventiveness!

I finished this relationship for several reasons but first and most importantly, I did not feel right with God. I was compromising myself and feared I was becoming a sex-object. This partnership was not in accordance with my relationship with God. I wanted a marriage truly made in heaven and what man was going to offer this to me?

At present I am celibate and that is fine – I do believe we need celibacy for certain periods in our lives although I would not necessarily advocate it permanently. There are alternative ways of touching and having contact with other people – by massage or complementary therapies such as reflexology or shiatsu just to name a few. I always enjoy having my hair brushed and many hairdressers now offer head massage as part of their services.

Dildos and other sex aids are easily purchased at Ann Summers shops on many high streets and the taboos which used to surround masturbation have now largely disappeared from our society. It should be remembered that there are more women than men in the population as a whole and therefore there are bound to be many single women, but there is no reason why they should not have sexual pleasure in today's world.

PS. I have recently met a lovely man many years younger than me who really likes me and he again has helped me in so many practical ways – improving my flat and making the garden beautiful. He has a good eye for design and is also talented in carrying out his ideas in a practical fashion. He also has a spiritual side and although there is a great difference in our ages, for the moment he is all I could wish for. Let the future unfold as it desires …

Chapter 11

'Recovery' written by Emma Harding

Many people who feel they may be experiencing mental health problems may wish to know when they might 'get better', or how they might start the process of recovery. Mental health services and service users have often had very different ideas about the subject, with service users sometimes rejecting the teams and medications that may not holistically address spiritual or other human needs that arise from the aftermath of often profound experiences, through lack of knowledge or resources.

Community mental health teams in the UK are based around the care programme approach with specific workers allocated to each client to maintain contact and co-ordinate their care, through developing implementing and reviewing care plans based on thorough needs assessment. This 'care programme approach' or CPA has been the dominant model in the UK, and is often driven by team members closely allied to the medical model of mental distress – that 'symptoms' such as hearing voices can be explained using the same concepts and language as physical health problems ('chemical imbalances' being a favourite). However a new philosophy is rapidly gaining ground – that of the recovery model.

The recovery model is based on the idea that service users themselves should indicate what their goals for 'recovery' should be – whether it be being able to join a local sports club or to write a book – and services are learning to incorporate these goals into the treatment plans for individual clients. The approach involves individuals developing relapse and crisis plans – based on their own experience of what works, so the people and practices that suit them best (such as who to feed the cat, which hobbies to continue to help the individual through) might be mobilised when symptoms return or look as if they are about to. These plans are developed in conjunction with mental health services, and may include 'advanced directives' – documents outlining which medications to use or avoid in case of involuntary admission to hospital, as well as other service-level arrangements.

An important facet of the recovery model is its focus on the individual's empowerment and involvement in directing their own recovery. This is enriched by the central tenet of valuing each story of recovery, through written, pictorial and spoken expressions of individuals' journeys. Listening to or reading different stories may help people wishing to improve aspects of their lives to find inspiration, motivation and ideas as to how to do this and it is argued that being aware of many different threads of the rich tapestry that is 'recovery' helps people weave their own understanding of their experience in a naturalistic way – very different from the experience of being told what your problems and solutions are in a clinical consulting room by someone you may not feel could not thoroughly understand the totality or details of a life-changing experience that they have not had.

One final point to bear in mind is that recovery is never total or complete and does not just refer to mental health problems. Everybody is recovering from or to something, whether it be a life event such as a wedding or a sense of severe alienation through mental health related discrimination. It may be dangerous to view yourself a 'recovered', with nowhere left to go, but after all, the journey, rather than arriving at the destination is often the more telling and important part of any adventure.

Chapter 12

Direct Payments

Following on from Emma's chapter on recovery, I would like to add a few paragraphs about Direct Payments and the way that they can aid recovery and empower the user.

As a result of a botched operation in 2003 I became unable to do any physical work and of course that included housework. I decided to employ a lovely Ukrainian lady to help in the house and this was costing me about £24 a week. Then a friend who was a social worker told me about Direct Payments. This is government money which has been made available to help disable people and carers have more control over their lives. A social worker from my Community Mental Health Team visited me at home and eventually the money to pay my cleaning lady became available and a separate account was set up at my bank to pay this lady. I give her a cheque each week when she comes and transforms my flat!

Recently I was asked to do a talk about my experience of Direct Payments to a meeting which included social workers, carers and mental health workers, to raise awareness of Direct Payments. One of my fellow speakers was also bi-polar and is an artist making screen-printed t-shirts. He talked about his experience of receiving a Creative Direct Payment to help him with the cost of art materials etc. I am now in the process of applying for one myself to cover the cost of printing cards from my paintings and for canvases etc. I also learned at this meeting that I could apply for a one-off Direct Payment for a new lap-top – this one being nearly worn out in the writing of this book!

It is obvious that this government initiative is a great step forward in the recovery process as it enables users to make choices about their future and to assist in empowering them to realise their dreams.

In 2011 the Recovery College at Springfield Hospital was opened, the first of its kind in the country. The college offers free courses to service users on a variety of subject ranging from 'Living with Mood Swings' to 'Introduction to Mindfulness' and 'Exploration of Spirituality in Recovery' and many more.

There are now recovery colleges in Kingston-on-Thames and other parts of South London.

Chapter 13

The Future of Mental Health

On October 20th 2007 I had the privilege of visiting the new Phoenix Unit for long-stay patients at Springfield Hospital in South London where I worked for a total of thirteen years, starting in 1976 as Patients' Librarian.

The new Unit was opened in September 2005 and is home to eighteen patients, both male and female. The architect who designed the unit, Karen Flatt, consulted patients and other interested parties such as the advocate throughout the building work and several patients told me how much they liked living in this new environment, which replaced a very run-down Victorian ward without a garden.The general appearance as you approach the Phoenix Unit is of a pleasant low-level Scandinavian-type building made partly of wood and partly of brick. On entering the unit which is secure, you have an impression of a hotel reception behind glass and curving corridors leading on the one side to the male bedrooms and on the other to the female rooms. The whole interior is made of light wood and the paintwork is conducive to a calm atmosphere. In fact the Advocate at Springfield who was consulted about the planning told me the number of complaints

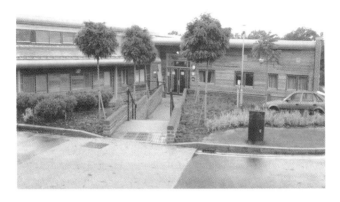

The new Rehabilition Ward at Springfield Hospital.

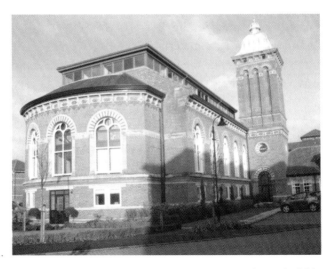

The former ballroom at Parkside Psychiatric Hospital, Macclesfield, Cheshire – now converted into luxury appartments.

from patients on Phoenix has dropped to virtually zero since the new building was opened.

I was shown round the unit by the ward Manager, who kindly allowed me to take photographs. Each patient has their own room comprising a bedsitter with sofa and bed and TV and en-suite bathroom with shower etc. There are also a laundry-room, occupational therapy room, kitchen for teaching cookery, communal dining room and psychology room and the whole is built round an enclosed courtyard garden which is well-planted. There are various therapies on offer such as music therapy, aromatherapy and massage, dance and drama therapies and frequent outings to the cinema and other places of interest.

Karen Flatt, the architect, told me the planning permission process was lengthy and involved both English Heritage and the Wandsworth Society as the hospital is located in the Borough of Wandsworth. Concerning building materials, the roof is made from western red cedar and the floors are made from bamboo which is very robust – the patients did not want carpets as they stain easily. The doors are all veneered. The users were consulted about colour schemes and I noticed a lot of mauve walls which are very calming.

In my opinion this building is an example of best practice for the future for long stay patients and evidence is already showing that patients do better in this type of environment. Hopefully other hospital trusts will recognize the need for real consideration of patients' needs in the future.

The whole question of physical environment is crucial when looking at the needs of mental health patients.

When the Care in the Community programme was introduced in the 1980's the idea of re-housing users in hostels and supported houses in the community was introduced. Fundamentally this was good thinking, provided it was implemented in the right way and there was still adequate in-patient provision in hospital if these patients needed more care for a while. Unfortunately in many areas hospitals were completely closed and users were not given proper long term support after, in many cases, having spent years in hospital and often becoming institutionalised to the extent that they could barely manage in the community. However some hospital trusts managed the transition well and the quality of life for these users vastly improved.

During the 80's I regularly visited service-users at two half-way houses in Streatham in the London Borough of Wandsworth, as part of my brief as a member of the Chaplaincy Team based at Springfield Hospital. Here two very large and imposing houses facing Tooting Bec Common were bought for the long term care of patients from Springfield.

No 4, a beautiful house built during the thirties is staffed by residential social workers, so there is always someone available if there is a crisis. Next-door at no 3 the users live independently but can always call on no 4 if they need any help from professionals. The atmosphere in these houses is very much like a family home with all the different personalities living under one roof and generally fairly amicably, although of course as in any family there can be crises and difficulties but generally life proceeds as normal. It must be so different for the residents from the old hospital regime and is to be encouraged wherever possible. I still visit from time to time and I am always given a warm welcome and a cup of tea and I count some of these people as personal friends – they care for each other, particularly at the unstaffed residence, and it is good to see people often moving on to independent living in their own flats.

This question of integrating patients with long term illness into the community is a difficult one and largely depends on the degree of severity of the illness but I know of long term schizophrenics who live independently and maintain a relatively comfortable way of life with the support of professionals and medication and of course other users and supportive family and friends.

I now carry out some voluntary art work with some of the residents of a privately-run care home for people with long-term mental health issues. This home is another example of best practice. The manager is extremely competent and a trained nurse, as well as being very hands-on with all the residents and welcomes help and suggestions concerning any improvements that can enhance the lives of those in her care. The cuisine is carried out by a qualified chef and the well appointed rooms (with en-suite showers and toilets and kettles for tea and coffee making) are furnished by Ikea. Obviously homes of this quality are few and far between but such high standards of care and accommodation should be the aim of local authority care-homes in the future.

I believe there will, sadly, be a greater need for child psychologists and other professionals in the future as society breaks down and the pressures of everyday life particularly in the cities. Already we are seeing an increase in drug-induced psychoses and depression in children. I do not believe prescribing anti-depressants to children is the answer. We have to take a deeper look at the root causes and use more hands-on therapies such as art therapy and complementary medicine to enable these sensitive children to regain their interest in life and improve their confidence.

I firmly believe that the syllabus for training psychiatrists should include a detailed module on complementary medecine and more research should be done into the benefits of, for example, massage for mental health users. Already research has shown that reflexology given on a regular basis can reduce the need for anti-depressants in women.

Furthermore it appears that long term use of psychiatric drugs can result in ME, depriving users of vital energy and zest for life.

We live in a 'chemical' age where the large pharmaceutical companies have a vested interest in producing more and new drugs for use in psychiatry – not always to the advantage of the patients who can suffer severe side-effects and can frequently be over-medicated. When I worked as an advocate during the nineties the most frequent problem that patients brought to our service was concern over the side effects of medication. Inappropriate weight gain and tremors were only two of the many unwanted side-effects of the prescribed drugs.

As I have mentioned above I believe there should be a radical rethink about the training of psychiatrists

– away from the tunnel-vision idea that drugs are the only way of dealing with those suffering mental distress – a more holistic approach would avoid the frequent over-prescribing and consequent added suffering for those already distressed. Complementary medicine could be offered alongside allopathic treatment and more 'talking therapies' would alleviate the need for so much medication. This vision can surely only reduce the enormous financial cost of drugs to the NHS and be more beneficial for those receiving it.

In a recent 'Woman's Hour' feature on BBC Radio 4 on mental health the Mental Health Foundation representative said that Primary Care Trusts should be applying for more funds for psychological therapists – there are only 3,000 trained and we need 10,000. One in four families in the UK has a member with mental health problems. She suggested that there should be more support for users in the Job Centres and more training for GP's in this area. There should be a shift in emphasis to more early intervention by professionals. A good example of this is taking place at Springfield Hospital in South London where their award-winning Early Intervention Service focuses on people aged 17 to 30 who have been experiencing the symptoms of psychosis for the first time. Studies have shown that with sustained treatment, over 80% individuals achieve symptomatic remission from a first episode of psychosis within six months.

Chapter 14

Laughter – the Best Medicine

In all the books I have read about mental health there is very little mention of that great healer – laughter. That is not to say it is absent from psychiatric wards – on the contrary some of my most humerous experiences have taken place on the ward, but it tends to be forgotten or lost amongst the medical jargon, advice on drugs and psychotherapy in books on mental health. In fact the only recollection of it, I have in my reading, is Freud's book entitled *On Jokes*.

It is a medical fact that the very physical act of laughing produces a change in the body chemistry and whenever I have had what I would call 'a great laugh' it feels as though the whole area around my stomach has been massaged – surely not a bad thing? And, of course, it improves our mood.

My best friend, Anne, used to hold 'Games Night' on a Monday, at her home in South-West London – in order to qualify to attend one had to have been a patient at the local psychiatric hospital. We would play 'Pictionary' and other board games and these gatherings were very popular and well-attended. They provided an opportunity for sometimes depressed or marginalised people to enjoy a light-hearted evening where you were completely accepted and valued and friendships deepened and flourished because of Anne's hospitality. I remember one particular evening we were laughing so much I wet my knickers – but it was worth it for the experience of sharing a joke!

It is worth remembering that some of our best-loved comedians have suffered with mood swings and I recall the amazing and original humour of Tony Hancock, who suffered terrible bouts of depression, and of course the zany Spike Milligan, a self-confessed sufferer from bi-polar disorder. Then coming more up-to date the exhuberant Ruby Wax, who has brought acceptance of mental illness into the so-called 'celebrity' arena.

I recently watched again the great 1970's film *One flew over the Cuckoo's Nest* with Jack Nicholson and co, where the inmates, led by Nicholson, stage a hilarious but believable 'take-over' of the asylum. The awakening of the idea that it is possible to escape from the drug-induced lethargy of the general psychiatric ward is played out very convincingly by the cast and Nicholson's (Mac) constant battles with the haridan Nurse Ratchett is reminiscent of my own battles with staff who sometimes are little more than key-toting jailers, whose sole role seems to be to be warders of the door to freedom.

Having made this sweeping statement I hasten to add that there are gems amongst the nursing staff – men and women who genuinely care for and engage with the patients in order to help them leave the ward and continue their recovery in the community.

So, to conclude, I would recommend a sense of humour as being a primary requisite for those entering a psychiatric ward, however depressed you feel, join in with others equally afflicted, to try and see the funny side of your situation and maintain a certain sense of proportion about things – we have been there and, thankfully, most of us have survived.

PS: This book would not have been published without my aunty Freda's generosity. She has also enabled me to finally leave London and fulfil my long-held wish to move to Brighton, which has been my place of refreshment and replenishment during the difficult times. I recommend a day at the seaside for any one needing uplifment of spirits and energy. Sea-bathing or any immersion in water is healing and life-giving!